I0786860

ISBN: 9798678724663

7-Day Diet

For Men

Metric Edition

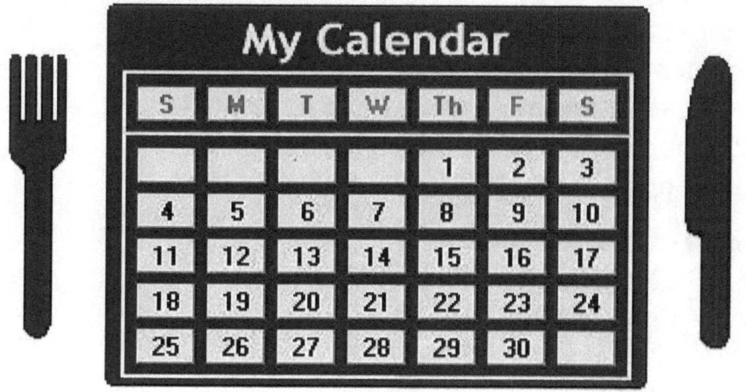

Gail Johnson, M.S. & Ronald Hill, Jr.

NoPaperPress™

CONTENTS

Being overweight or obese matters. Excess weight puts excessive strain on your body. Studies have shown that overweight people have a greater risk of serious illness than those who are slimmer – and the greater the degree of overweight the greater the risk. People who are overweight are more susceptible to certain illnesses, especially heart and circulatory diseases, type-2 diabetes, as well as gallbladder and liver disorders. Being overweight also has a negative impact on self esteem and appearance. Whereas, those who have successfully lost weight report a sense of well-being – both physically and mentally – and a well-deserved pride in their achievement.

To millions of people losing weight has become not only a aspiration but almost a way of life. The fact that so many have found it difficult to realize their goal has fostered a flood of fad-diet books. Some of the diets insist that it's not how much you eat but the combination of foods, or the type of food you eat that's important. Most exclude forbidden (but often nutritious and reasonably low calorie) foods. Others are big on motivation and offer hand-holding emotional support but little else. In fact, almost every diet book on the market is devoid of hard facts, real data, analysis and insight.

What Makes a Good Weight-Loss Diet?

Every good weight-loss diet must have the following three characteristics:

1) A good diet must provide you with an understanding of weight control as well as the knowledge you need to reduce your weight to the desired level.

2) A good diet must help you remain healthy while you are losing weight.

3) A good diet must lead you to a healthier way of eating and exercising that will, in the long term, help you keep off the weight you have lost.

The weight-loss diet featured in this eBook is the so-called "balanced diet;" i.e., a diet that is not only low calorie and reasonably low in fat, but is also nutritionally balanced. The *7-Day Diet*, however, does not meet all the criteria set forth above.

While you will get some "dieting insight" and some idea of how much you can eat and still lose weight, you will not get a real understanding of weight control. That's not its purpose. What you do get in this eBook is a healthy diet – and a diet that if followed will promote weight loss. Think of the *7-Day Diet* as a quick fix, a healthy jump start, that will get you going on the right track – but it is not the long-term answer.

Knowledge is Required for Long-Term Success

Long-term success is not about finding the "right" diet. It's about developing both an understanding and a plan that will result in healthier eating and physical activity habits. Without a doubt identifying the behaviors that have contributed to your eating more calories than your body needs is important, very important. But assuming you are successful in determining why you overeat, what do you do next?

The truth is that weight control, although a relatively complex issue, is governed by a set of logical, scientific principles, and the acceptance and understanding of these principles – augmented of course by desire and self-discipline – can lead you to sure and lasting weight management. Most health professional agree that losing weight sensibly and safely requires a multifaceted approach that includes setting reasonable weight-loss goals, changing eating habits, and getting adequate exercise. The desire to lose weight and the discipline to start and stay on a weight-control program are crucial. But along with desire and discipline, it is our belief that **only an in-depth understanding of weight control, nutrition and exercise will lead to long-term success**. As is true with many complex subjects, to achieve you need more than rules – you need information and a solid grasp of the subject.

For a complete weight control discussion, a through understanding and the guidance you need to succeed in the long term we recommend you read, *Weight Control - Metric Edition* by Vincent W. Antonetti, Ph.D., an eBook also published by NoPaperPress.

When to Use the 7-Day Diet

1) If you're in weight maintenance mode but notice your weight creeping up. You want to stop the upward trend and lose a few pounds as well. Here's the perfect solution: Use the *7-Day Diet for Men* to quickly lose a few unwanted kilos!

2) You've let your weight get out of control. So you decide to go on a diet. It doesn't matter what diet, or how much weight you want to

lose. Your first move should be to go on the *7-Day Diet for Men,* lose a quick 1 to 2 kilos and get on the right track. After the 7-Day Diet does its job, you can switch to a longer-term diet.

Begin With a Medical Exam

Before you begin any weight loss program you should know where you stand, i.e., your current health status. Assessing your current status in areas such as cardio (aerobic) capacity, body-fat, and even how appropriate your nutritional practices are, will help you establish what you should emphasize in your weight control program and help you set goals. For a comprehensive health self assessment we refer you once more to *Weight Control - Metric Edition* by Vincent W. Antonetti.

Everyone should at the very least have a medical assessment, or exam, before starting a weight loss diet. Why? You need to make sure your health will allow you to lower your caloric intake and increase your physical activity. The medical checkup may be as simple as a visit to a physician who is familiar with your medical history, or it may be a thorough physical exam. The physician conducting the medical exam should be made aware of and should approve the specific weight loss diet you're planning. Additionally, if you are going to engage in some sort of physical activity in conjunction with this diet and especially if you have been totally inactive, or if you have or suspect you have cardiovascular disease or other health problems, or if you are obese, or if you are 40 or older, before embarking on the physical fitness portion of your weight control program you should have a stress test supervised by a physician.

What's in the 7-Day Diet eBook?

This eBook actually contains two 7-day diets: a 1500 kcalorie diet, and for even faster weight loss a 1200 kcalorie diet. Both diets have a meal plan (menu) for each and every day. And every day features a "Recipe and Diet Tip of the Day."

Which Calorie Level is Right for You?

- **1200 kcalorie Diet:** Smaller men, older men and inactive men should select the 1200 kcalorie diet.

- **1500 kcalorie Diet:** Larger men, younger men and active men should choose the 1500 kcalorie diet.

How Much Weight Will You Lose?

Weight loss occurs when your food energy intake is less than the total energy you expend. This difference in calories is referred to as your <u>calorie deficit</u>. How much weight you lose depends on the magnitude of your calorie deficit.

People on any weight-loss diet invariably want to know how much weight they will lose – and how fast. Simple metabolic calculations make a rough estimate possible. Physiologists have long known that to lose one pound requires a deficit of approximately 7700 kcalories. Therefore, if a person's total kcalorie deficit over time is known, their weight loss over time can be calculated.

Consider an overweight 40 year-old male, who is approximately 1,78 m tall and weighs 84 kg, is relatively inactive, and consumes about 3000 kcalories per day. (In other words, this overweight man is eating about 3000 kcalories per day to maintain his weight at 84 kilos, that is to neither gain nor lose weight.)

Now, if this statistically average man goes on a 1200 kcal reducing diet, his daily deficit would be 3000 – 1200 = 1800 kcalories. Recall that to lose one kilogram of body weight requires a deficit of approximately 7700 kcalories. In 7-days, therefore, this man's deficit would be 1800 kcalories per day x 7 days = 12600 kcalories, and he should lose 126000 / 7700, or 1,6 kilos. If instead the man in our example selected the 1500 kcalorie diet, he would lose slightly more, about 1,4 kilos in 7 days.

But at the start of any diet there is also considerable water loss. When this water loss is accounted for, **on the 7-Day Diet, most men lose 2 to 2,5 kilos** – depending on whether the 1200 or 1500 kcalorie diet is selected. Smaller men, older men and less active men will lose a bit less and larger men, younger men and more active men often much more.

Exactly how much weight you will lose depends on how much you weigh, your age and your activity level. Again, for the full story see *Weight Control - Metric Edition* by Vincent W. Antonetti, Ph.D.

Lose Weight Even Faster - Exercise

Our bodies are just not built to be immobile and passive. The sad fact, however, is that after years of education and information programs by government agencies, medical associations and insurance companies,

relatively few Americans engage in regular planned exercise – despite the reality that we need to be active to keep our systems working efficiently and rid ourselves of emotional tension. Moreover, exercise burns calories, speeds up your metabolism and is an invaluable part of any weight control program. There are two ways to become more physically active: 1) Increase the physical activity in your daily life; and 2) Start on a regular exercise program. Better still would be a combination of both.

Simply stated there are three basic types of exercise: aerobic, stretching, and strengthening.

Aerobic exercises (also called "cardio") condition your cardiovascular system. Aerobic exercises, such as jogging, swimming, cycling, brisk walking, skipping rope, and many others, are typically deep breathing and continuous, with rhythmic and repetitive contractions of your large muscle groups. The trait most aerobic exercises have in common is that they make you work hard and require you process a great deal of oxygen.

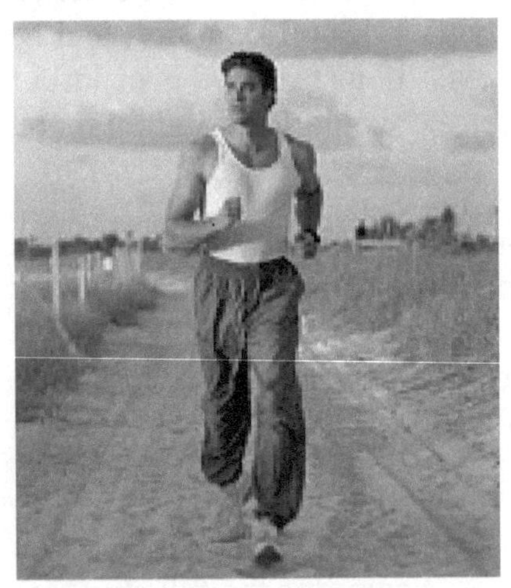

Some typical aerobic exercises are: Most strenuous include bicycling, cross-country skiing, dancing (aerobic), hiking in rugged terrain, ice hockey, jogging, jogging in place, rowing, skipping rope, stair climbing, and stationary cycling. Somewhat less strenuous are basketball, field hockey, calisthenics, handball, racquetball, skiing (downhill), soccer, squash, tennis (singles), volleyball, and walking (briskly). Least strenuous aerobic exercises consist of badminton, baseball, bowling, croquet, dancing, gardening, golf (carrying or pulling clubs), horseback riding, housework, ping-pong, shuffleboard, softball, tennis (doubles) and walking (moderate to leisurely).

Stretching-type exercises such as yoga, tai chi, Pilates and to a lesser extent calisthenics can improve your flexibility – and some of the exercises can make you somewhat stronger.

As you age you inevitably start to loose flexibility. Your gait becomes stiffer; you can't stand quite as upright as you used to; it becomes tougher to bend over; and you have difficulty turning your neck. Regardless of your age, however, stretching can make you more flexible, less injury prone, and can reduce the pain and discomfort associated with tight muscles and shortened tendons. Realize, however, that stretching exercises do not condition your heart and lungs. Stretching exercises are fine as long as they are performed in addition to rather than in place of an aerobic exercise.

Most experts do recommend stretching before and after an aerobic or strength routine. However, never stretch cold muscles and always do some form of warm up prior to stretching. Stretch slowly and hold gently. You should stretch to the point of feeling a mild pull, but you should never feel pain. And when you stretch – do not bounce.

Muscle building and strengthening exercises, e.g., weight lifting, use of the machines found in fitness centers and isometrics.

Once more, as you age you loose muscle mass, your bone density decreases and you lose strength. Exercises like weight lifting strengthen your muscles, bones and joints. Strengthening exercises also reduce your risk of developing osteoporosis, a severe bone-loss disease, which can lead to easily fractured bones and all the complications that often follow. Strong muscles not only allow you to lift a sleepy four-year old out of a car without difficulty and lug groceries up to a second floor apartment, but as with increased flexibility, strong muscles also make you less injury prone. Moreover, because **muscle uses many more calories than fat, when you replace fat with muscle, your metabolism actually speeds up.**

For everything you need to know about exercise see *Exercise Smart - Metric Edition,* an eBook by Earl Simmons also published by NoPaperPress.

Guidelines for Healthy Eating

No single food can supply all the nutrients you need in the amounts you need. The most important factors in nutrition are variety, variety, variety! **Variety is the key to a nutritious diet.** As a means of setting strategies for food selection, the U.S. Department of Health and Human Services and the Department of Agriculture issue Dietary

Guidelines every five years. The 2005 Dietary Guidelines describe a healthy diet as one that:

1) Emphasizes fruits, vegetables, whole grains, and fat-free or low-fat milk products.
2) Includes fish, poultry, lean meats, beans and nuts.
3) Is low in saturated fats, trans fats, cholesterol, salt (sodium) and added sugars.

The guidelines encourage adults to consume a variety of nutrient-dense foods and beverages within their caloric needs. In 2005, the afore mentioned U.S. government agencies recommended how much should be eaten from each of the basic food groups (i.e., from the fruit group, vegetable group, grains group, meat and beans group, milk group, and oils group) to meet your caloric goal – whether you are trying to lose weight or maintain weight. All this information and more can be found in the eBook *Eat Smart - Metric Edition* published by NoPaperPress.

Even though most adults can get all the vitamins and minerals they need by merely consuming a variety of nutritious foods (from the fruit group, the vegetable group, the grains group, the meat and beans group, the milk group, and the oils group), many physicians recommend a daily multi-vitamin/mineral supplement – just in case you don't eat the way you should.

Be aware that some micronutrients, such as the fat-soluble vitamin A, can be harmful if taken in large quantities. To be safe your multi-vitamin/mineral supplement should contain no more than 100 percent of the recommended dietary allowance (RDA) for each vitamin or mineral. Generally, you don't need the high doses in multi-vitamin/mineral supplements labeled "therapeutic" or "extra-strength." There may be medical reasons for taking larger amounts of a vitamin or mineral than the RDA provides, but check with your doctor first. For example, adults over age 50 and vegetarians who do not eat animal foods may be advised to get their vitamin B_{12} from a supplement or from fortified foods. Men with limited exposure to sunlight may need a vitamin D supplement, and individuals who seldom eat dairy products or other rich sources of calcium may need to take a calcium supplement.

As you age, adequate protein intake and body protein reserves are more important than ever, especially during times of emotional and physical stress. Body proteins are constantly being made and used during your lifetime to maintain the functions of the cells and organs, and protein is needed to help to prevent muscle loss. Good sources of protein-rich foods are meats, fish, eggs, dairy products, dried beans and peas, and soy products.

Vitamin B_{12} can be a problem nutrient for older adults. Vitamin B_{12} enables your body to manufacture healthy red-blood cells and assists in the transmission of electrical signals between nerve cells. The acid in your stomach helps release vitamin B_{12} from the protein in the food you eat. This must occur before vitamin B_{12} is absorbed in your intestines. But as you age, the amount of stomach acid you produce decreases. Less hydrochloric acid lessens the amount of vitamin B_{12} separated from proteins in foods and can result in poor absorption of vitamin B_{12}. Vitamin B_{12} is found naturally in meat, fish, poultry, eggs and fortified cereals. But recent studies have revealed that up to 30 percent of adults aged 50 years and older may also have atrophic gastritis, an increased growth of intestinal bacteria, that renders them unable to normally absorb vitamin B_{12} in food. They are, however, able to absorb the synthetic vitamin B_{12} added to fortified foods and dietary supplements. As a result, fortified foods and vitamin supplements may be the best sources of vitamin B_{12} for adults 50 years and older.

In fact the newest U.S. Modified Food Guide Pyramid for Adults over 70 recommends that this age group take a dietary supplement for vitamin B_{12}, calcium and vitamin D. (Vitamin D supplements are particularly important for older adults with limited exposure to sunlight.)

7-Day Diet Breakfast Guidelines

You've heard it before. It's important to start the day right and eat breakfast. **So try to allow time for breakfast before you rush off to work.** If need be do some preliminary preparation the night before such as setting up your coffee maker, deciding on and measuring the amount of cereal you will be eating, etc. Many busy people prepare breakfast at home and bring it to work in a plastic container. Do what you need to do – but don't skip breakfast!

In the *7-Day Diet for Men,* you may substitute wholesome **whole-grain cereal** for any specified cereal. So feel free to substitute Weetabix for Shredded Wheat, Oatibix for Cheerios, etc. And if you don't like the scrambled egg called for on Day 5, have a hard-boiled egg or make a fried egg instead. Maybe the cantaloupe called for in the meal plan is not in season. No problem. Just replace the cantaloupe with a half cup of orange juice. For a more complete list of food substitutions and exchanges see the text and table on pages 14 and 15.

7-Day Diet Mid-Day Meal Guidelines

Most days the *7-Day Diet for Men,* lunch is either soup or a sandwich.

Feel free to substitute a soup you favor in place of those indicated – provided the basic type of soup and calorie counts are similar to those specified in the *7-Day Diet for Men.* For example, Day 1 calls for a cup of Lentil Soup (140 kcalories), but if you prefer, you may substitute a cup of Bean Soup – which is in the same food group as lentil soup and contains approximately the same calorie count.

Warm Weather Substitutions: On warm and especially very hot days, you may want to substitute a sandwich, or a tuna or salmon salad for the soup of the day.

7-Day Diet Dinner Guidelines

On the *7-Day Diet for Men,* one of the dinner mainstays is a "Tossed Green Salad." Prepare your "Tossed Green Salad" in a bowl with a volume of at least 16 ounces, or 2 cups. First add about 1 cup of either green leaf lettuce, Romaine lettuce or a mesclun mix. Then add, as desired, half cup of green veggies such as broccoli, celery, cucumber, peppers, spinach, or watercress. This vegetable combination will, on average, total about 35 kcalories. You will be eating a "Tossed Green Salad" just about every day at dinnertime. Remember that variety is the key to a nutritious diet. So be sure to vary the ingredients of the salad.

Top your "Tossed Green Salad" with <u>2 tablespoons (30 ml) of any light salad dressing</u> available at your local supermarket that contains no more than 50 kcalories for 2 tablespoons (30 ml). Some of our favorite light salad dressings are:

Ken's Steakhouse Fat Free Raspberry Pecan
Kraft Light Done Right House Italian
Newman's Own Lighten Up! Balsamic Vinaigrette
Wishbone Just 2 Good Honey Dijon

Your "Tossed Green Salad" with 30 ml (2 tablespoons) of salad dressing will cost you roughly 70 kcal but will be packed with lots of health-giving vitamins, minerals and fiber.

Snack Guidelines

On Some of the menus in the *7-Day Diet for Men* feature a morning snack, an afternoon snack and an evening snack. The main snacks are:

Yogurt: We recommend Dannon Light at 90 kcalories per container (at this writing). Select any flavor. There are other brands you may prefer but whatever you buy be certain you eat no more than 90 kcalories worth of yogurt for your snack.

Fresh Fruit in season: Choose an apple, pear, peach, plum, watermelon (1 cup), etc. You will be eating fruit every day. So vary the fruit that you select to get good array of micronutrients.

Handful of Unsalted Mixed Nuts: Nuts and seeds are loaded with protein and fiber. This eBook uses a "handful" as a convenient descriptor rather than something like "16 almonds = 100 kcalories," but be aware that although nuts are a healthy food, nuts are also a high-calorie food. Buy mixed nuts to get a range of micronutrients. And please no salt.

Popcorn: Popcorn is a tasty, nutritious high-fiber, filling snack. For a busy adult you can't beat Orville Redenbacher's Smart Pop Popcorn Mini Bag which you can just nuke in your microwave and eat.

But for the best popcorn we suggest you purchase a hot-air popper which uses popping corn, a type of corn that bursts from the kernel and puffs up when heated. (A popular brand is Orville Redenbacher's Original Gourmet Popping Corn.) A hot-air popper will make a large batch of popcorn in a few minutes. For a snack, eat only a one liter bowl of the popcorn and store the remainder for another day. At this writing, you can purchase a good hot-air popper for approximately € 20.

About Bread

First understand that bread, more specifically whole-grain breads, are good sources of complex carbohydrates and dietary fiber, as well as several B vitamins (thiamin, riboflavin, niacin, and folate), vitamin E, and minerals (iron, magnesium and selenium).

In recent years, however, sliced bread loaves have gotten larger, as have the bread slices inside these loaves. Just a few years ago the standard slice of bread contained about 70 kcalories – now most are 100 plus kcalories.

The *7-Day Diet* requires whole-grain bread at no more than 70 kcalories per slice. Quite a few bakers sell thin sliced or "light" sliced bread. The difficult part is finding a whole grain thin sliced or "light" bread (with about 70 kcalories per slice). Whatever the brand, make sure the first word in the Ingredients list is "whole." "Pepperidge Farm Small Slice 100% Whole Wheat" is a good choice. It's whole grain, has 70 kcalories per slice and it tastes good too.

Exchanging & Substituting Foods

If there is a food listed in the *7-Day Diet* that you don't like, or perhaps that you forgot to pick up while shopping, you probably can exchange or substitute another food in its place – a technique used by dieticians. Exchanging a food listed in a diet for another food with approximately equal caloric value and nutritional content is the foundation of a successful long-term diet. Substitution possibilities are almost endless but have to be done carefully.

The easiest substitutions are those within the same food group, such as exchanging one vegetable variety for another, or a glass of milk for a cup of yogurt. More sophisticated exchanges cross food groups, for instance replacing 100 g of turkey with a tablespoon of peanut butter spread on a piece of whole wheat bread. Both foods are complete protein and both contain about 175 kcalories.

Refer to the calorie table in Appendix A (at the end of this eBook). With some understanding and experience, you can use this table to help you substitute foods called for in the *7-Day Diet* with equal calorie foods from the same food group.

Breakfast: You may substitute any cereal for any other wholesome cereal. For example, if you're not crazy about having Shredded Wheat for breakfast on Day 7, substitute Wheat Chex or Cheerios, etc. If you don't like the soft-boiled egg called for on Day 2, make yourself a scrambled egg instead. And if Cantaloupe is on the menu but is not in season, replace the cantaloupe with half an orange or half cup of orange juice.

Snacks: Again, where yogurt is specified you may substitute an equivalent volume of skim milk, but to maintain a nutritionally balanced diet keep this snack a dairy selection. Similarly, when fruit is on the agenda, you may select another type of fruit but do not stray from the fruit group. Nuts and popcorn can be interchanged at will. (Incidentally, we recommend you buy a hot-air popper.)

7-Day Facts

As mentioned previously, there are, two diet plans in this eBook: 1200 kcalorie Diet and a 1500 kcalorie diet. Both diets have a detailed meal plan for each of the 7 days. In addition, there is also a "Recipe of the Day" and "Diet Tip of the Day".

7-DayFood Item	Substitute
Artichoke salad (Day 4)	Any green veggie for artichokes
Asparagus, green beans, etc	Any other green veggie
Brown rice	Medium potato
Cantaloupe (½)	Orange juice (120 ml)
Cereal	Exchange with any other whole-grain cereal
Chicken Sausage	Chicken or turkey franks
Chocolate (Day 6)	2 small sugar cookies or 4 graham cracker squares
Cod (Day 6 recipe)	Any other white fish
Cottage cheese (1 cup)	250 ml skim milk (probably impractical)

Eggs	Egg Beaters Egg Substitute
Fresh fruit in season	¾ cup canned fruit (no sugar added)
Frozen entrée (Day 5)	Frozen entrée with same calorie count
Grapefruit (½)	Orange (medium)
Handful of mixed nuts	Popcorn Mini Bag
Pancakes (Day 3 recipe)	Kashi Go Lean Waffles
Pasta sauce (Day 7 recipe)	Bottled Marinara tomato sauce
Peanut butter	Almond butter
Popcorn	Handful of mixed nuts
Pork chop	Poultry or fish (125 g)
Raisin bread	Plain whole-grain bread
Salmon (Day 1 recipe)	Tuna
Soup	Any soup with same calorie count
Tossed green salad	Unlimited steamed greens (spinach, broccoli, etc)
Turkey	Chicken (white meat)
Veggie burger (Day 2 recipe)	Any other type of non-meat burger
Whole-grain bread	Vary bread type (whole wheat, rye, etc)
Wine (120 ml)	Grapes (1 cup)
Yogurt	180 ml skim milk

Food Substitution Chart

Both the 1200-kcalorie and 1500-kcalorie diets adhere to the United States Department of Agriculture recommendation that suggest a balanced diet should have approximately 50 percent of its calories from carbs, about 20 percent from protein sources and 30 percent or less from fat.

1200-kcalorie Diet: Due to the relatively low calorie level, you will just barely get all the nutrients and micro nutrients you need – and you also might feel hungry at times.

1500-kcalorie Diet: You will easily get all the nutrients and micro nutrients you need from 1500 kcalories. And most men do not feel hungry at this calorie level.

Important Notes

1) Coffee or tea may be decaf or regular brew. If desired, skim milk and a sugar substitute may be added to coffee or tea.
2) Fried eggs, scrambled eggs, or an omelet should be cooked in a pan coated with a non-stick cooking spray.
3) On bread, corn on the cob, baked potatoes, if desired, you may use a zero-calorie butter substitute spray.
4) Cereals should be whole grain and preferably unsweetened. At the top of the list are Old-fashioned Oat Meal, Wheatena and Weetabix. Among other reasonably healthy choices are Cheerios, Wheat Chex, Wheaties, some Kashi cereals and Farina.
5) Bread may be either plain or toasted whole grain, such as whole wheat, whole rye or pumpernickel. If desired, bread may be sprayed with a zero-calorie butter substitute.
6) Use only lean cuts of meat trimmed of all visible fat. Poultry should be limited to chicken or turkey breasts (white meat only and skinless).
7) When canned tuna or salmon is specified, use only fish packed in water.
8) An unlimited amount of green salad may be eaten, but the salad dressing should be as specified. (Incidentally, in the meal plans Evoo means extra virgin olive oil.)
9) Use freely as desired: clear unsweetened coffee, clear unsweetened tea, water, seltzer water and any diet soda.
10) Use freely as desired: clear soups without fat, bouillon, and seasonings such as mustard, cinnamon, dill, herbs, red and black pepper, curry, vinegar, lemon juice and sections, and dill and sour pickles.
11) Any specified snack may be moved to any other part of the day, and/or combined with breakfast, lunch or dinner.

Keeping It Off

Within five years, more than 90 percent of all dieters regain every kilo they have lost. Why? In most cases it's because after losing weight most people eventually revert to their pre-diet eating and exercising habits, and this inevitably leads to their regaining the weight they lost– and often more. The fact is the less you weigh, the less you need to eat to sustain your lower weight.

A study, published in a 2005 issue of the Annals of Internal Medicine, that followed 4,000 people for three decades suggests that in the long term, 90 percent of men and 70 percent of women will become overweight. Interestingly, half of the men and women in the study, who had made it well into adulthood without a weight problem, ultimately also became overweight and a third actually became obese. The point being that you can never become complacent. You must continually watch your weight because we are all at risk of becoming overweight.

As mentioned previously, the key to long-term weight control success is knowledge and understanding, combined of course with desire and self-discipline.

7-Day Step-Up Maintenance Plan

This is a method used by some successful maintainers. After you lose weight at a known calorie level, you step up to the next higher calorie level to try to determine your weight maintenance calorie level.

For example, Roger Griffin a 1,8 m, relatively inactive 58 year old, went from 89 kilos to 81 kilos on a 1500 kcalorie per day plan. (He used our *30-Day Quick Diet for Men – Metric Edition* also published by NoPaperPress.) He then stepped up to the 1800 kcalorie per day plan and after 14 days discovered he was still losing weight, albeit at a much slower rate. But he didn't want to lose more weight, so he stepped up to 2100 kcalorie per day where his weight did not change. He had found his approximate weight maintenance calorie level (2100 kcalories), i.e., the number of calories he could eat without gaining or losing weight.

How to Use This eBook

First, depending on your size, your age and how active you are, refer to page 7 and choose the diet calorie level that's right for you, either 1200 or 1500 Calories per day.

- **1200-kcalorie Meal Plan starts on page 25.** (See page 21 for the applicable Food Shopping List.)

- **1500-kcalorie Meal Plan starts on page 31.** (See page 22 for the applicable Food Shopping List.)

Next, study the meal plan for the calorie level you have selected and then scan the appropriate Food Shopping List. Finally, using the food shopping list prepare a list of the foods you don't have on hand– that you will need to buy.

Food Shopping List (1200-kcal Diet)

Orange juice (1 liter)
Orange (1)
Cantaloupe (1)
Banana (1)
Fresh fruit in season (apple, peach,
plum, etc) (8)
Fresh or frozen blueberries (1 package)
Wheaties (2 servings)
Cheerios(1 serving)
Shredded Wheat (1 serving)
Eggs (2)
Pancake
syrup (lite)
Coffee and or Tea
Skim milk (1 liter)
Yogurt (120 g nonfat, any flavor) (3)
Whole grain bread (7 slices)
Hot dog bun (1)
Hamburger bun (1)

Tomatoes (2), Summer Squash,
Zucchini, Peas Green beans, Asparagus
(7 spears), Beets (3 small) Brown Rice

Tomato Bouillon, Beef Bouillon

Turkey (sliced white meat) (25 g)
Ham (sliced & lean) (50 g)
Swiss Cheese (low-fat) (50 g)
Cottage cheese (250 ml low fat)
Tuna (solid white albacore packed in water) (75 g can)

Salmon (100 g to 125 g fillet)
Cod (100 g to 125 g fillet)

Veal chop (100 g oz, lean)
Chicken sausage (2 links about 70 g per link)
Lean Cuisine Thai-Style Chicken (Café Classics™)
Whole wheat Pasta (225 g serves 4 people)
Salad ingredients (See page 13 for recommended salad dressings)
Popcorn (see pages 13 &14), Unsalted Nuts (3 handfuls), Dark Chocolate (25 g)

Note: For additional food items see Day 1 - Day 7 Recipes.

Food Shopping List (1500-kcal Diet)

Orange juice (1 liter)
Orange (1)
Cantaloupe (1)
Banana (2)
Fresh fruit in season (apple, peach, plum, etc) (9)
Fresh or frozen blueberries (1 package)

Wheaties (2 servings)
Cheerios (1 serving)
Shredded Wheat (1 serving)
Eggs (2)
Pancake syrup (lite)
Coffee & tea
Skim milk (2 liters)
Yogurt (120 g nonfat, any flavor) (5)
Whole grain bread (14 slices)
Hot dog bun (1)
Hamburger bun (1)

Tomatoes (2), Summer Squash, Zucchini, Peas,
Green beans, Asparagus (7 spears), Beets (3 small)

Vegetable Bouillon, Beef Bouillon

Turkey (sliced white meat) (25 g), Turkey bacon (2 slices)
Ham (sliced & lean) (50 g)
Swiss Cheese (low-fat) (75 g)
Cottage cheese (1 cup low fat)
Tuna (solid white albacore packed in water) (75 g can)
Salmon (100 to 125 g fillet)
Cod (100 to 125 g fillet)

Veal chop (100 g, lean)
Chicken sausage (2 links about 70 g per link)
Lean Cuisine Thai-Style Chicken (Café Classics™)
Whole wheat Pasta (225 g serves 4 people)
Salad ingredients (See page 13 for recommended salad dressings)
Popcorn (see pages 13 &14), Unsalted Nuts (5 handfuls), Dark
Chocolate (25 g),
Small Cookies and Biscuits

Note: For additional items see Day 1 - Day 7 Daily Menus & Recipes.

1200 kcal DAILY MENUS

DAY 1 – 1200 kcal Meal Plan

BREAKFAST	Calories	Totals
Cantaloupe (½ medium)	50	
Wheaties (30 g) + 120 ml skim milk + ½ banana	190	
Coffee (See page 19.)	10	250 kcal

MORNING SNACK		
Coffee or tea	10	10 kcal

LUNCH		
Lentil soup (1 cup = 240 ml)	140	
Turkey (30 g) on 1 slice of rye bread	115	
Lettuce & tomato slices	20	
Skim milk (½ cup = 120 ml)	40	315 kcal

AFTERNOON SNACK		
Coffee or tea	10	10 kcal

DINNER		
Baked salmon with salsa (Day 1 Recipe page 41)	215	
Summer squash, zucchini and tomatoes	60	
Brown rice (½ cup = 100 g)	100	
Tossed green salad w 30 ml low-cal dressing*	70	
Fresh fruit in season (apple, peach, plum, etc)	70	
Water	0	515 kcal

* See page 15.

EVENING SNACK		
Popcorn – no butter (1 liter bowl)	80	
Coffee or tea	10	90 kcal
		1190 kcal

DAY 2 – 1200 kcal Meal Plan

BREAKFAST	Calories	Totals
Orange juice (½ cup = 120 ml)	50	
Soft-boiled egg	80	
Whole wheat toast (1 slice) (See page 16.)	70	
Coffee	10	210 kcal
MORNING SNACK		
Coffee or tea	10	10 Cal
LUNCH		
Tuna salad: 90 g tuna, 5 ml oil, onion & celery	175	
Lettuce & tomato wedges	20	
Rye bread (1 slice)	65	
Fresh fruit in season – (apple, pear, peach, etc)	70	
Coffee or tea	10	340 kcal
AFTERNOON SNACK		
Yogurt (6 oz – nonfat, any flavor)	90	
Coffee or tea	10	100 Cal
DINNER		
Veggie burger – (1 patty) (Day 2 Recipe - page 42)	100	
Low-fat cheddar cheese (1 thin slice)	50	
Seeded hamburger roll	140	
Tossed green salad with 30 ml = 2 Tbsp low-cal	70	
Beets (3 small size)	45	
Fresh fruit in season (apple, peach, plum, etc)	70	
Skim milk (150 ml)	60	535 kcal
EVENING SNACK		
Coffee or tea	10	10 kcal
		1205 kcal

<u>DAY 3</u> – 1200 kcal Meal Plan

BREAKFAST	**Calories**	**Totals**
Orange juice (½ cup = 120 ml)	50	
Wild blueberry pancakes (Day 3 Recipe - page 43)	190	
Light syrup (1 Tbsp = 15 ml)	30	
Coffee	10	280 kcal
MORNING SNACK		
Coffee or tea	10	10 kcal
LUNCH		
Peanut butter (30 g) on 2 slices bread	330	
Skim milk (1 cup = 240 ml)	90	
Fresh fruit in season (apple, peach, plum, etc)	70	490 kcal
AFTERNOON SNACK		
Coffee or tea	10	10 kcal
DINNER		
Vegetable bouillon	0	
Broiled pork chop (1 cm thick & trimmed of fat)	260	
Green peas (75 g)	55	
Tossed green salad w 30 ml low-cal dressing	70	
Water with lemon section	15	400 kcal
EVENING SNACK		
Coffee or tea	10	10 kcal
		1200 kcal

DAY 4 – 1200 kcal Meal Plan

BREAKFAST	Calories	Totals
Fresh sliced orange	75	
Cheerios (30 g) + 120 ml skim milk + 15 raisins	190	
Coffee	10	275 kcal

MORNING SNACK		
Fresh fruit in season (apple, peach, plum, etc)	70	
Coffee or tea	10	80 kcal

LUNCH		
Cottage cheese – low fat (1 cup = 225 g)	180	
Tossed green salad with 2 Tbsp = 30 ml low-cal	70	
Small whole-grain roll	80	
Hot or iced tea	10	340 kcal

AFTERNOON SNACK		
Handful of unsalted mixed nuts	100	
Coffee or tea	10	110 kcal

DINNER		
Grilled chicken sausage (2 links 70 g per link)	180	
Artichoke-bean salad (Day 4 Recipe - page 44)	190	
Green beans - steamed	25	
Water	0	395 kcal

EVENING SNACK		
Coffee or tea	10	10 kcal
		1210 kcal

<u>DAY 5</u> – 1200 kcal Meal Plan

	Calories	Totals
BREAKFAST	**Calories**	**Totals**
Cantaloupe (½ medium)	50	
Scrambled egg	80	
Whole-wheat toast (1 slice)	70	
Coffee	10	210 kcal
MORNING SNACK		
Yogurt (¾ cup = 120 g) – nonfat, any flavor	90	
Coffee or tea	10	100 kcal
LUNCH		
Split pea soup (1 cup = 240 ml)	150	
Tomato slices & chopped fresh basil and 1 tsp =	60	
Whole-grain bread (1 slice)	65	
Hot or iced tea	10	285 kcal
AFTERNOON SNACK		
Coffee or tea	10	10 kcal
DINNER		
Frozen Chicken Dinner (See page 45.)	300	
Tossed green salad with 2 Tbsp = 30 ml low-cal	70	
Fresh fruit in season (apple, peach, plum, etc)	70	
Water	0	440 kcal
EVENING SNACK		
Two small sugar cookies	150	
Coffee or tea	10	160 kcal
		1205 kcal

DAY 6 – 1200 kcal Meal Plan

BREAKFAST	Calories	Totals
Orange juice (½ cup = 120 ml)	50	
Fried egg	80	
Whole-wheat toast (1 slice)	70	
Coffee	10	210 kcal

MORNING SNACK		
Yogurt (¾ cup = 120 g) – nonfat, any flavor	90	
Coffee or tea	10	100 kcal

LUNCH		
Vegetable soup (1 cup = 240 ml)	110	
Grilled cheese sandwich (2 slices 2% cheese)	240	
Pickle spears	0	
Water	0	350 kcal

AFTERNOON SNACK		
Fresh fruit in season (apple, peach, plum, etc)	70	
Coffee or tea	10	80 kcal

DINNER		
Baked Herb-Crusted Cod (Day 6 Recipe - page 46)	230	
Asparagus (about 7 spears cooked & drained)	20	
Tossed green salad with 30 ml low-cal dressing	70	
Water	0	320 kcal

EVENING SNACK		
Dark chocolate (25 g)	150	
Coffee or tea	10	160 kcal
		1220 kcal

DAY 7 – 1200 kcal Meal Plan

BREAKFAST	Calories	Totals
Orange juice (½ cup = 120 ml)	50	
Shredded Wheat (50 g) + 120 ml skim milk + ½	260	
Coffee	10	320 kcal

MORNING SNACK		
Coffee or tea	10	10 kcal

LUNCH		
Beef bouillon – unlimited amount	0	
Bologna (60 g) w mustard on 2 slices rye bread	280	
Pickle spears	0	
Diet soda or water	0	280 kcal

AFTERNOON SNACK		
Yogurt (¾ cup = 120 g) – nonfat, any flavor	90	
Coffee or tea	10	100 kcal

DINNER		
Pasta w Marinara sauce (Day 7 Recipe - page 47)	225	
Tossed green salad with 30 ml low-cal dressing	70	
Fresh fruit in season (apple, peach, plum, etc)	70	
Italian or French bread (1 slice)	80	
Water with lemon section	15	460 kcal

EVENING SNACK		
Coffee or tea	10	10 kcal
		1180

1500 kcal DAILY MENUS

DAY 1 – 1500 kcal Meal Plan

BREAKFAST	kcal	Totals
Cantaloupe (½ medium size)	50	
Wheaties (30 g) + 120 ml skim milk + ½ sliced	190	
Whole wheat toast (1 slice) **(See page 15.)**	65	
Coffee **(See page 19.)**	10	315 kcal

MORNING SNACK		
Fresh fruit in season (apple, peach, plum, etc)	70	
Coffee or tea	10	80 kcal

MID-DAY MEAL		
Lentil soup (1 cup = 240 ml)	140	
Turkey (30 g) on 1 slice of rye bread	115	
Lettuce & tomato slices	20	
Skim milk (½ cup = 120 ml)	40	315 kcal

AFTERNOON SNACK		
Two small oatmeal raisin cookies – or equivalent	160	
Coffee or tea	10	170 kcal

EVENING MEAL		
Baked salmon with salsa **(Day 1 Recipe - page 41)**	215	
Summer squash, zucchini and tomatoes	60	
Brown rice (½ cup = 100 g)	100	
Tossed salad with 30 ml low-cal dressing	70	
Fresh fruit in season (apple, peach, plum, etc)	70	
Water	0	515 kcal

EVENING SNACK		
Popcorn – no butter (1 liter bowl)	100	
Coffee or tea	10	110 kcal
		1505 kcal

<u>DAY 2</u> – 1500 kcal Meal Plan

BREAKFAST	kcal	Totals
Orange juice (½ cup = 120 ml)	50	
Soft-boiled egg	80	
Whole wheat toast (2 slices)	130	
Coffee	10	270 kcal

MORNING SNACK		
Yogurt (¾ cup = 6 fl oz = 120 g) – nonfat, any flavor	90	
Coffee or tea	10	100 kcal

MID-DAY MEAL		
Tuna salad: 90 g tuna, 1 tsp = 5 ml oil, onion & celery	175	
Lettuce & tomato wedges	20	
Rye bread (1 slice)	65	
Fresh fruit in season – (apple, pear, peach, etc)	70	
Coffee or tea	10	340 kcal

AFTERNOON SNACK		
Handful of unsalted mixed nuts	100	
Coffee or tea	10	110 kcal

EVENING MEAL		
Veggie burger – (1 patty) **(Day 2 Recipe - page 42)**	100	
Low-fat cheese (1 slice) plus lettuce, tomato &	90	
Seeded hamburger roll	100	
Beets (3 medium size)	55	
Tossed salad with 30 ml = 2 Tbsp low-cal dressing	70	
Fresh fruit in season (apple, peach, plum, etc)	70	
Skim milk (¾ cup = 180 ml)	70	555 kcal

EVENING SNACK		
Sorbet – any flavor (½ cup = 120 ml)	120	
Coffee or tea	10	130 kcal
		1505 kcal

DAY 3 – 1500 kcal Meal Plan

BREAKFAST	kcal	Totals
Orange juice (½ cup = 120 ml)	50	
Wild blueberry pancakes **(Day 3 Recipe - page 43)**	190	
Bacon (2 slices)	90	
Low-calorie syrup (1 Tbsp = 15 ml)	30	
Coffee	10	370 kcal

MORNING SNACK	kcal	Totals
Yogurt (¾ cup = 120 g) – nonfat, any flavor	90	
Coffee or tea	10	100 kcal

MID-DAY MEAL	kcal	Totals
Peanut butter (30 g) on 2 slices of bread	330	
Skim milk (1 cup = 240 ml)	90	
Fresh fruit in season (apple, peach, plum, etc)	70	490 kcal

AFTERNOON SNACK	kcal	Totals
Carrot sticks w 60 g low-fat cottage cheese & chives	60	
Coffee or tea	10	70 kcal

EVENING MEAL	kcal	Totals
Vegetable bouillon – unlimited amount	0	
Broiled pork chop (1 cm thick – trimmed of fat)	265	
Green peas (75 g)	55	
Tomato-cucumber salad (30 ml low-cal dressing)	70	
Water	0	390 kcal

EVENING SNACK	kcal	Totals
Popcorn – no butter (1 liter bowl)	70	
Coffee or tea	10	80 kcal
		1500 kcal

DAY 4 – 1500 kcal Meal Plan

BREAKFAST	kcal	Totals
Fresh sliced orange	75	
Cheerios (30 g) + 120 ml skim milk + 15 raisins	190	
Whole wheat toast (1 slice)	65	
Coffee	10	340 kcal

MORNING SNACK	kcal	Totals
Fresh fruit in season (apple, peach, plum, etc)	70	
Coffee or tea	10	80 kcal

MID-DAY MEAL	kcal	Totals
Cottage cheese – low fat (1 cup = 225 g)	180	
Tossed green salad with 30 ml = 2 Tbsp low-cal	70	
Small whole-grain roll	80	
Hot or iced tea	10	340 kcal

AFTERNOON SNACK	kcal	Totals
Handful of unsalted mixed nuts	100	
Coffee or tea	10	110 kcal

EVENING MEAL	kcal	Totals
Grilled chicken sausage (2 links 70 g per link)	180	
Artichoke-bean salad **(Day 4 Recipe - page 44)**	190	
Green beans – steamed, unlimited amount	25	
Whole-wheat bread (1 slice)	65	
Water with lemon section	15	475 kcal

EVENING SNACK	kcal	Totals
Two small sugar cookies – or equivalent snack	150	
Coffee or tea	10	160 kcal
		1505 kcal

DAY 5 – 1500 kcal Meal Plan

BREAKFAST	kcal	Totals
Grapefruit (½ medium size)	75	
Scrambled egg	80	
Bacon (2 slices)	90	
Whole-wheat toast (1 slice)	65	
Coffee	10	320 kcal

MORNING SNACK		
Yogurt (¾ cup = 120 g) – nonfat, any flavor	90	
Coffee or tea	10	100 kcal

MID-DAY MEAL		
Split pea soup (1 cup = 240 ml)	150	
Tomato slices & chopped basil and 2 tsp = 10 ml	100	
Whole-grain bread (1 slice)	65	
Hot or iced tea	10	325 kcal

AFTERNOON SNACK		
Handful of unsalted mixed nuts	100	
Coffee or tea	10	110 kcal

EVENING MEAL		
Frozen Chicken Dinner **(See page 45)**	300	
Tossed green salad with 30 ml low-cal dressing	70	
Whole-grain bread (1 slice)	70	
Fresh fruit in season (apple, peach, plum, etc)	70	
Water with lemon section	15	525 kcal

EVENING SNACK		
Crackers or biscuits – any brand	120	
Coffee or tea	10	130 kcal
		1510 kcal

<u>DAY 6</u> – 1500 kcal Meal Plan

<u>BREAKFAST</u>	<u>kcal</u>	<u>Totals</u>
Orange juice (½ cup = 120 ml)	50	
Wheat Flakes (30 g) + 120 ml skim milk + ½	190	
Whole-wheat toast (1 slice)	65	
Coffee (See note on page 15.)	10	315 kcal

<u>MORNING SNACK</u>		
Fresh fruit in season (apple, pear, peach, etc)	70	
Coffee or tea	10	80 kcal

<u>MID-DAY MEAL</u>		
Vegetable soup (1 cup = 240 ml)	110	
Turkey breast (25 g) on 1 slice rye bread	105	
Lettuce & tomato slices	20	
Glass of skim milk (¾ cup = 180 ml)	60	295 kcal

<u>AFTERNOON SNACK</u>		
Two small chocolate chip cookies – or equivalent	140	
Coffee or tea	10	150 kcal

<u>EVENING MEAL</u>		
Baked Herb-Crusted Cod (Day 6 Recipe - page 46)	230	
Spinach (65 g) steamed with small amount of	100	
Asparagus (7 spears cooked & drained)	20	
Baked potato (medium size)	100	
Whole grain bread (1 slice)	65	
Water with lemon section	15	530 kcal

<u>EVENING SNACK</u>		
Sorbet – any flavor (½ cup = 120 ml)	120	
Coffee or tea	10	130 kcal
		1500 kcal

<u>DAY 7</u> – 1500 kcal Meal Plan

	kcal	Totals
BREAKFAST		
Orange juice (½ cup = 120 ml)	50	
Shredded Wheat (50 g) + 120 ml milk + ½ banana	260	
Coffee	10	320 kcal
MORNING SNACK		
Handful of unsalted mixed nuts	100	
Coffee or tea	10	110 kcal
MID-DAY MEAL		
Beef bouillon – unlimited amount	0	
Bologna (60 g) w mustard on 2 slices rye bread	280	
Pickle spears	0	
Diet soda or water	0	280 kcal
AFTERNOON SNACK		
Yogurt (¾ cup = 120 g) – nonfat, any flavor	90	
Coffee or tea	10	100 kcal
EVENING MEAL		
Pasta with Marinara sauce **(Day 7 Recipe - page 47)**	225	
Tossed green salad with 30 ml low-cal dressing	70	
Fresh fruit in season (apple, peach, plum, etc)	70	
Italian or French bread (1 medium-thick slice)	80	
Glass of red wine (120 ml)	100	
Water with lemon section	15	560 kcal
EVENING SNACK		
Crackers or biscuits – any brand	120	
Coffee or tea	10	130 kcal
		1500 kcal

RECIPE & DIET TIPS

<u>Day 1 - Recipe</u>

<u>Baked Salmon with Salsa</u>

This is a simple, straight-forward recipe. The advantage of a simple recipe is there are no hidden calories.

4   150 g salmon fillets
6   Tbsp (90 ml) bottled tomato-pepper salsa

Brown salmon fillets in non-stick pan and place in baking dish. Put fillets in an oven preheated to 175 °C for about 10 minutes.

Plate the salmon. Stir prepared tomato-pepper salsa and spoon it over the salmon.

<u>Serves 4</u>. One salmon fillet is about 215 kcal.

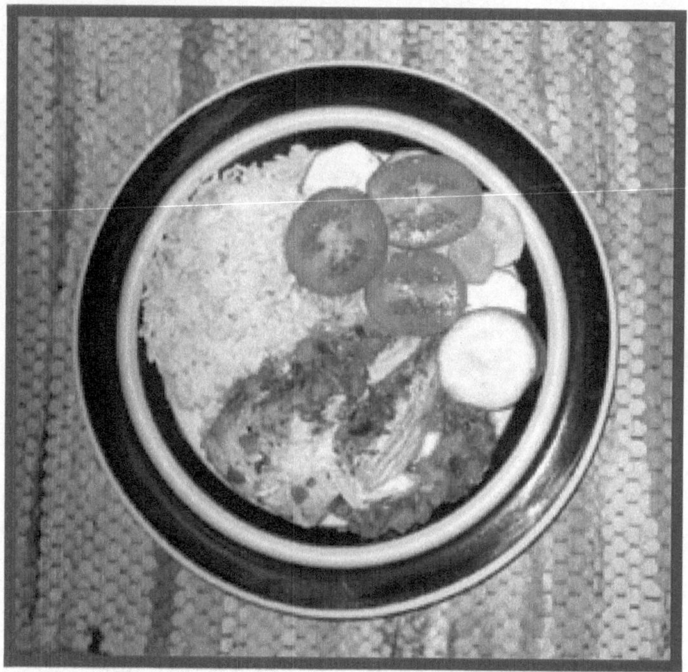

<u>**Diet Tip of the Day:**</u> **Have soup more often.** Most <u>non-cream-based</u> soups are filling and low-calorie.

Day 2 - Recipe

Veggie Burger

In many countries, vegetable-based burgers can be purchased at a local supermarket. The veggie burger can be made from vegetables, soy, nuts, mushrooms, textured vegetable protein, dairy, or a combination of these foods.

Two popular veggie burgers in the UK are Fry's Range Burger and Alicer Range Burger. Fry's Burger is made chiefly from soy protein and wheat gluten. Other countries have similar products.

To prepare, follow package directions. The version shown below has an added slice of low-fat cheddar cheese. The lettuce, tomato and ketchup shown actually add very few extra calories.

The veggie burger patty plus low-fat cheese and a seeded amounts to about 290 kcal.

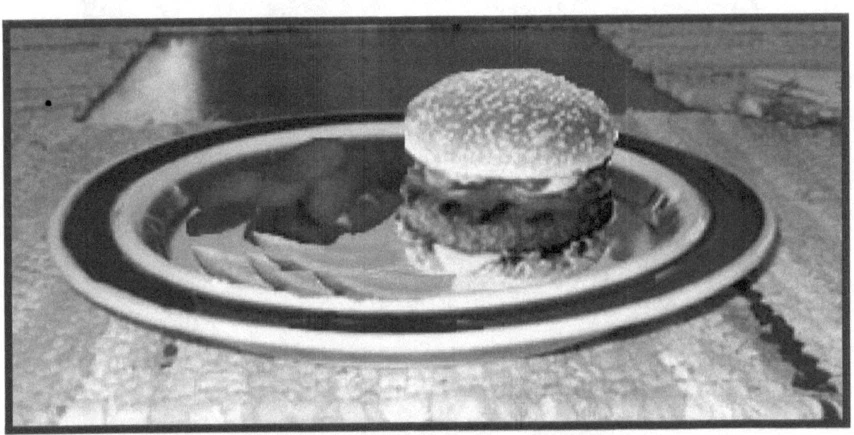

Diet Tip of the Day: **Drink lots of water** – about 8 glasses per day. Add a slice of lemon to make it more interesting. Often, when you think you're hungry, you are just thirsty. So, next time you head for a snack, drink some water first and see if that does it for you.

<u>Day 3 - Recipe</u>

<u>Wild Blueberry Pancakes</u>

This recipe makes a relatively low calorie, wholesome batch of delicious wild blueberry-whole wheat-buttermilk pancakes.

125 g	whole-wheat flour
240 ml	buttermilk
1	egg
15 ml	(1 tablespoon) vegetable oil
10 g	(1 teaspoon) baking powder
5 g	(½ teaspoon) baking soda

Stir ingredients until blended. Add 100 g (¾ cup) blueberries and gently stir. Using medium heat, preheat a non-stick skillet coated with cooking spray. Pour slightly less than 60 ml (¼ cup) of batter onto skillet per pancake. Cook slowly until bubbles break on surface of pancake. Turn and cook until other side is lightly browned. Makes 8 pancakes.

Pictured below are wild-blueberry pancakes with two slices of bacon. <u>**Serves 4**</u>. Each pancake is about 95 kcal

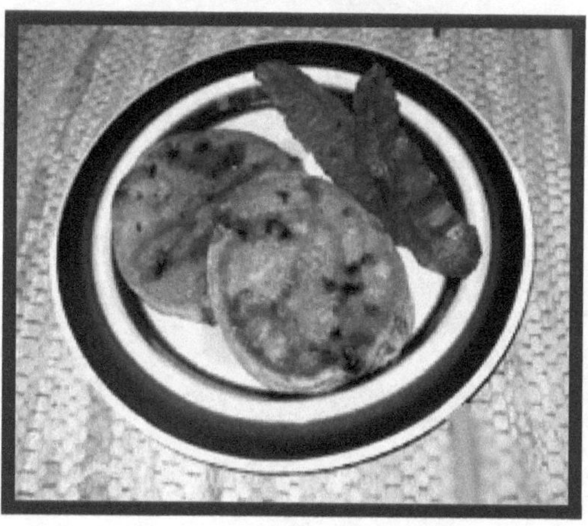

<u>**Diet Tip of the Day:**</u> A peanut butter sandwich on whole wheat bread with a glass of skimmed milk and an apple makes a nutritious, reasonably low-calorie lunch.

43

<u>Day 4 - Recipe</u>

<u>Artichoke-Bean Salad</u>

500 g	white kidney beans
10	artichoke hearts, quartered
⅓ cup	chopped oregano
⅓ cup	chopped parsley
3	cloves garlic, chopped
1	lemon, juiced

Combine ingredients in medium-size bowl. Stir in 60 ml (¼ cup) extra-virgin olive oil.   Salt and black pepper to taste.

<u>Serves 6</u>. Approximately 190 kcal per serving.

Pictured on the plate below are two grilled chicken sausage links with salsa, steamed green beans and the artichoke-bean salad. (Incidentally, this artichoke-bean combination over mixed salad greens served with a whole-grain bread makes a delicious, nutritious and reasonable low-calorie main course.)

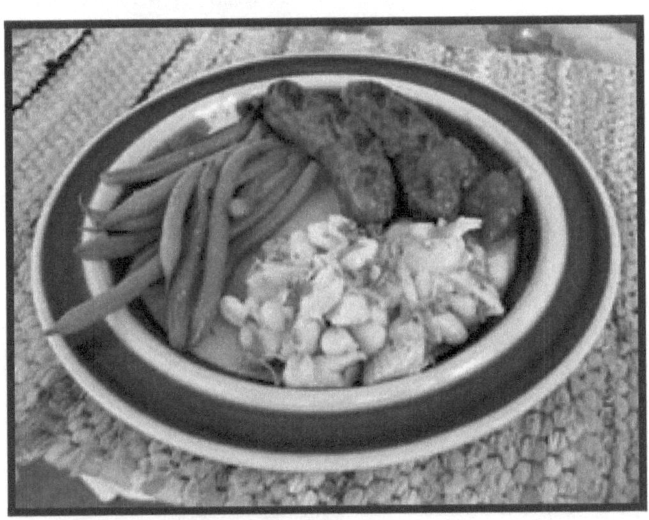

<u>Diet Tip of the Day:</u> Have a small meal before you go to a party. A hardboiled egg, an apple, and a thirst quencher (like water, tea, seltzer, or diet soda) will take the edge off your appetite and make it easier to resist the high-calorie goodies.

<u>Day 5 - Recipe</u>

No recipe today. The dinner for Day 5 is Lean Cuisine Sesame Stir Fry with Chicken (for the both the 1200-kcalorie diet and 1500-kcalorie diet).

In some instances, frozen may actually be better than fresh, because if you keep fresh fruit and vegetables in your fridge for a long time, they lose some of their nutritional value. Whereas, frozen foods are usually processed and packaged within hours of being picked. And the freezing process itself does not destroy nutrients. So buying frozen and then defrosting when you want the fruit or vegetable may actually be more nutritious.

According to the U.S. Department of Agriculture, food stored continuously at -17 °C or below is always safe to eat. Freezing keeps food safe and preserves food for extended periods because it prevents the growth of microorganisms that cause food spoilage and illness.

Please read the important Frozen-Food Safety Warning in Appendix B.

Use an appliance thermometer to monitor your freezer's temperature. If a refrigerator freezing compartment can't maintain -17 °C or if the freezer door is opened frequently, use it for short-term food storage, and eat those foods as soon as possible for best quality. Use a free-standing freezer set at -17 °C or below for long-term storage of frozen foods. Again, keep a thermometer in your freezing compartment or freezer to check the temperature.

Because freezing keeps food safe almost indefinitely, recommended freezer storage times are to preserve quality (taste, etc) of food, not the safety or nutritional value. **The quality of frozen dinners or entrees in a freezer at -17 °C will be maintained for 3 to 4 months.**

If there is a power outage, or if your freezer fails, or if the freezer door is left ajar by mistake, the food may still be safe to use. As long as a freezer with its door ajar continues to run, to cool, the foods should stay safe overnight. If a repairman is on the way or it appears the power will be restored soon, just keep your freezer door closed. A freezer full of food will usually keep about 2 days if the door is kept shut; a half-full freezer will last about a day. The freezing compartment of a refrigerator may not keep foods frozen as long. If the freezer is not full, group packages together to help maintain their low temperature.

During a power failure, you may want to put dry ice, a block or bags of ice in the freezer, or transfer foods to a friend's freezer until power returns. Again, use an appliance thermometer to monitor the temperature. To determine the safety of foods when the power goes on, check their condition and temperature. If food is partly frozen, still has ice crystals, or is as cold as if it were in a refrigerator (4 °C), it is safe to refreeze or use. It's not necessary to cook raw foods before refreezing. **If in doubt discard the food.And always discard frozen food whose temperature has exceeded 40 °F for more than two hours.**

Baked Herb-Crusted Cod

4   Cod fish fillets – 120 to 150 g each
2   tablespoons (Tbsp) flour (50 g)
2   Tbsp cornmeal (50 g)
2   Tbsp minced fresh herbs
2   teaspoons (tsp) lemon juice (10 ml)

Sprinkle cod with lemon juice. Mix flour, cornmeal and herbs and dust the cod with the cornmeal- herb mixture. Bake in oven at 190 °C for 10 minutes. Add salt and black pepper to taste.

Serves 4.   One serving is about 230 kcal (for cod only).

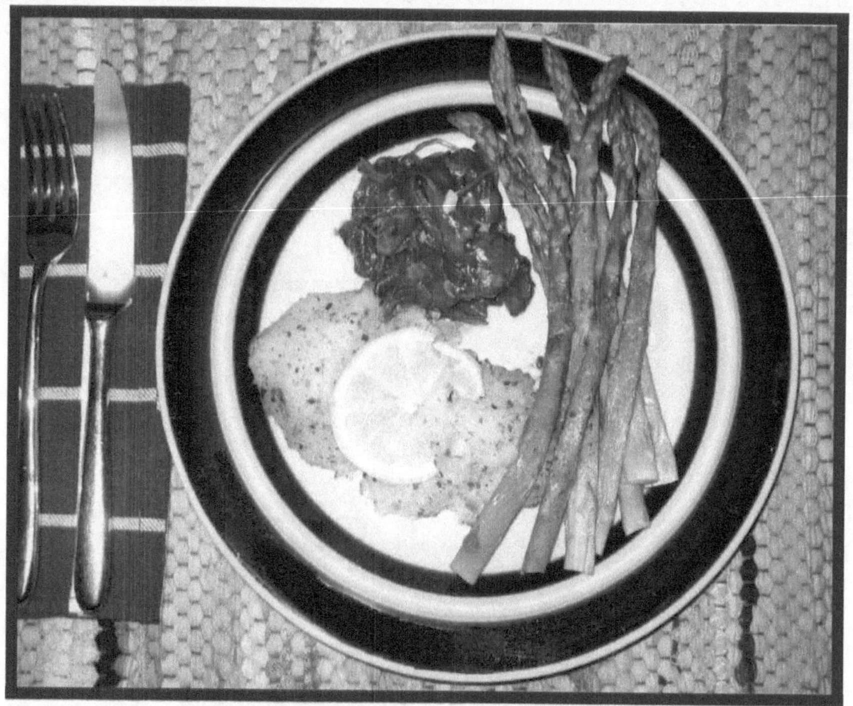

Diet Tip of the Day: **Take a daily multi-vitamin-mineral supplement.** This is very important when you're on a diet – as a kind of insurance policy.

Pasta with Marinara Sauce

Tomato sauce: Sauté ½ small onion, chopped fine, in 1 tsp (5 ml) olive oil. Add two finely chopped garlic cloves, 200 g chopped plum tomatoes and some chopped fresh oregano. Stir and cook about 5 minutes on a low flame. (If the tomato sauce is a bit too thick, dilute it with 60 ml of the liquid in which you cooked the pasta.)

225 g   whole-wheat pasta

The spiral pasta shape shown below is called Fusilli, and a is our favorite because all the pasta ridges really hold the sauce.

Bring two liters of lightly salted water to a boil. Add pasta and stir occasionally (to keep pasta from sticking to the bottom of the pot). Keep water boiling and cook until pasta are "al dente." (Cooking time is approximately 9 minutes.)

Drain pasta, add marinara sauce and serve hot.

Serves 4. One serving is about 225 kcal.

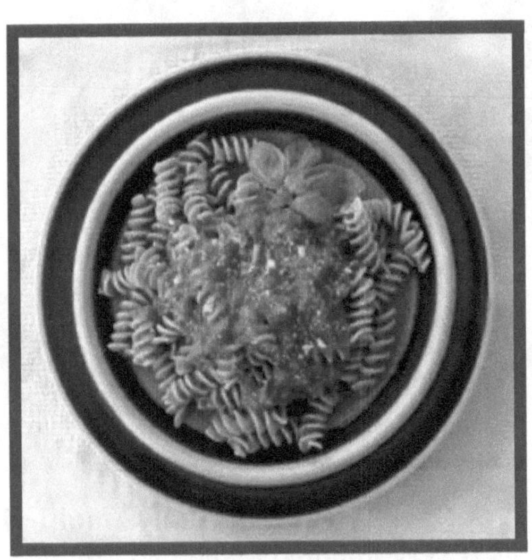

Diet Tip of the Day: **Beware of alcoholic beverages.** Beer has about 13 kcal per ounce, wine 25 kcal per 30 ml and whiskey 71 kcal per 30 ml.

Appendix B: Frozen-Food Safety

Increasingly, international food giants like ConAgra, Nestlé and others that supply many millions of people with processed foods concede that they cannot ensure the safety of their food products. Frozen foods pose a particularly serious safety problem because unsuspecting consumers buy frozen foods for their convenience and incorrectly believe that cooking frozen foods is a matter of taste – not safety.

Still the food industry says that extensive outbreaks of food-borne illness are rare, even though it is well-known that most of the millions of cases of food-borne illness every year go unreported or are not traced to the source. For example, each year approximately 40,000 cases of salmonella poisoning are reported in the United States – but perhaps as many as one million go unreported. (Salmonella is a type of bacteria most often found in poultry, eggs, unprocessed milk, meat and water.) Recently salmonella pathogens in some frozen meals have sickened thousands of people.

How could this happen? First, the supply chain for the ingredients in processed foods – from flour to fruits and vegetables to flavorings – is becoming more complex and global in the drive to keep food costs down. As a result, government and industry officials concede that almost every food ingredient is now a potential carrier of pathogens. A further complication is that a large number of food companies subcontract processing work to save money and don't require suppliers to test for pathogens. In fact, companies often don't even know who is supplying their ingredients.

In addition, many frozen-food manufacturers have stopped cooking their products at high temperatures, a tactic they call the "kill step," which is intended to eliminate any lingering microbes. Frequently this process step turns some of the frozen food ingredients into mush. So, instead the "kill step" has been shifted to consumers. For example, ConAgra has added food safety instructions to its frozen meals, including the Healthy Choice brand. A typical "frozen-food safety" instruction offers this guidance: "Internal temperature needs to reach 165°F (75°C) as measured by a food thermometer in several spots." Moreover, General Mills, now advises consumers to avoid microwaves altogether and cook their frozen pizzas only in a conventional oven.

Bottom line: To be safe, always cook frozen foods so that the internal temperature reaches 165°F (75°C) as measured by a good food thermometer.

100-Day Super Diet-1200 Calorie*	Weight Loss for Men - Metric*
100-Day Super Diet-1500 Calorie*	Maximum Weight Loss- 1200 Calorie*
100-Day No-Cooking Diet-1200 Cal*	Maximum Weight Loss- 1500 Calorie*
100-Day No-Cooking Diet-1500 Cal*	Weight Control - U.S. Edition
90-Day Smart Diet-1200 Calorie*	Weight Control - Metric. Edition
90-Day Smart Diet-1500 Calorie*	Professional Weight Control Women - U.S.
90-Day No-Cooking Diet - 1200 Cal*	Professional Weight Control Women -
90-Day No-Cooking Diet - 1500 Cal*	Professional Weight Control Men - U.S.
90-Day Perfect Diet - 1200 Calorie*	Professional Weight Control Men - Metric
90-Day Perfect Diet - 1500 Calorie*	Weight Maintenance - U.S. Edition*
60-Day Perfect Diet-1200 Calorie*	Weight Maintenance - Metric. Edition*
60-Day Perfect Diet-1500 Calorie*	Weight Maintenance - UK Edition
50-Day Flex Diet-1200 Calorie*	Weight Loss for Senior Men*
50-Day Flex Diet-1500 Calorie*	Weight Loss for Senior Women*
30-Day Quick Diet - for Women*	Eat Smart - U.S. Edition*
30-Day Quick Diet - for Men*	Eat Smart - Metric Edition
30-Day No-Cooking Diet*	Eat Smart - UK Edition
30-Day Diet for Women - Metric Ed	Exercise Smart - U.S. Edition
30-Day Diet for Men - Metric Ed	Exercise Smart - Metric Edition
25 Day Easy Diet-1200 Calorie*	Exercise Smart - UK Edition
25 Day Easy Diet-1500 Calorie*	Total Fitness - U.S. Edition
25-Day No-Cooking Diet	Total Fitness - Metric Edition
10-Day Express Diet	Total Fitness - UK Edition
10-Day No-Cooking Diet*	Total Fitness for Women-U.S. Edition*
7-Day Diet for Women*	Total Fitness for Women - Metric
7-Day Diet for Men*	Total Fitness for Women - UK Edition
7-Day No-Cooking Diets*	Total Fitness for Men - U.S. Edition*
90-Day Gluten-Free Diet-1200 Cal*	Total Fitness for Men- Metric Edition*
90-Day Gluten-Free Diet-1500 Cal*	Total Fitness for Men - UK Edition
30-Day Gluten-Free Quick Diet*	Senior Fitness - U.S. Edition*
30-Day Gluten-Free No-Cooking Diet*	Senior Fitness - Metric Edition*
7-Day Diet for Women - Metric	Senior Fitness - UK Edition*
7-Day Diet for Men - Metric	Computer Diet - U.S. Edition*
7-Day Gluten-Free Express Diet*	Computer Diet - Metric Edition*
7-Day Gluten-Free No-Cooking Diet*	Reliable Weight Loss - U.S. Edition
90-Day Vegetarian Diet-1200 Calorie*	Reliable Weight Loss - Metric Edition
90-Day Vegetarian Diet-1500 Calorie*	101 Weight Loss Tips*
30-Day Vegetarian Diet*	101 Healthy Eating Tips*
7-Day Vegetarian Diet*	101 Lifelong Fitness Tips*
Weight Loss for Women*	101 Weight Maintenance Tips
Weight Loss for Women - Metric	101 Weight Loss Recipes
Weight Loss for Women - UK	101 Gluten-Free Weight Loss Recipes
Weight Loss for Men*	101 Vegetarian Weight Loss Recipes*

* These titles are available as both ebooks and paperbacks.
NoPaperPress ebooks sold by Amazon, Apple, Google, Barnes & Noble and Kobo.
NoPaperPress paperbacks are only sold by Amazon.

www.ingramcontent.com/pod-product-compliance
Lightning Source LLC
Chambersburg PA
CBHW051419250726
48655CB00003B/1141